What Is Substance Use Disorder?

By Racquel Foran

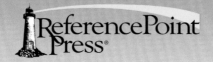

ReferencePoint Press®

San Diego, CA

3 9082 14208 9401

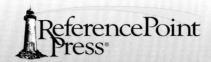

© 2021 ReferencePoint Press, Inc.
Printed in the United States

For more information, contact:
ReferencePoint Press, Inc.
PO Box 27779
San Diego, CA 92198
www.ReferencePointPress.com

Content Consultant: Jason Ramirez, Acting Assistant Professor, Department of Psychiatry and
Behavioral Sciences, University of Washington

LIBRARY OF CONGRESS CATALOGING-IN-PUBLICATION DATA

Names: Foran, Racquel, 1966- author.
Title: What is substance use disorder? / by Racquel Foran.
Description: San Diego : ReferencePoint Press, [2021] | Series: Teen disorders | Includes
   bibliographical references and index. | Audience: Grades 10-12
Identifiers: LCCN 2020003553 (print) | LCCN 2020003554 (eBook) | ISBN 9781682829554
   (hardcover) | ISBN 9781682829561 (eBook)
Subjects: LCSH: Substance abuse--Juvenile literature. | Substance abuse--Diagnosis--
   Juvenile literature. | Substance abuse--Treatment--Juvenile literature.
Classification: LCC RC564.3 .F67 2021 (print) | LCC RC564.3 (eBook) | DDC 362.29--dc23
LC record available at https://lccn.loc.gov/2020003553
LC eBook record available at https://lccn.loc.gov/2020003554

CONTENTS

From High Achiever to Substance User

Kate heard the car pull out of the driveway, so she knew her mom was gone. She rushed downstairs to confirm and then hesitated. She wondered whether she was really going to steal from her mom. But she already knew the answer. She needed money because couldn't face a full day of school without her drugs. She knew where to get them, but she would have to skip her first class to get the cash to pay for them. Kate would make a quick visit to the pawn shop to trade the necklace she had stolen for cash and then head to school.

The pawn shop didn't pay much, but it was enough to get her a few pills. She got them from a friend who had a prescription for Adderall for his attention-deficit/hyperactivity disorder (ADHD); he sold his pills instead of taking them. There were a few kids at school who sold prescription drugs. Most of them stole them from their parents a few pills at a time.

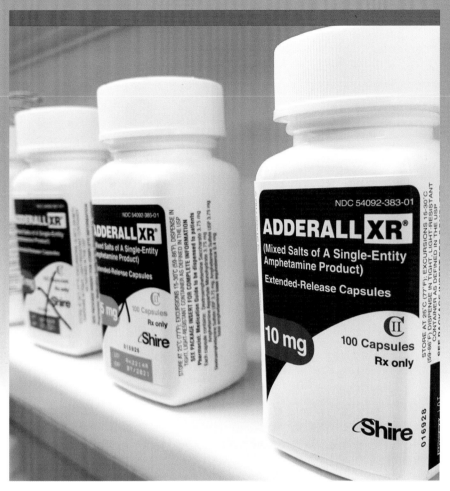

Some people use substances that are prescribed for another person. This can be very dangerous.

After getting the pills, it was a typical Tuesday for Kate. When she got home after school, she told her mom she felt a little tired and was going upstairs to have a nap. She really planned to take another pill to get her through a long evening.

A few minutes later, Kate's mom went to check on her. She found her daughter on the bedroom floor convulsing with

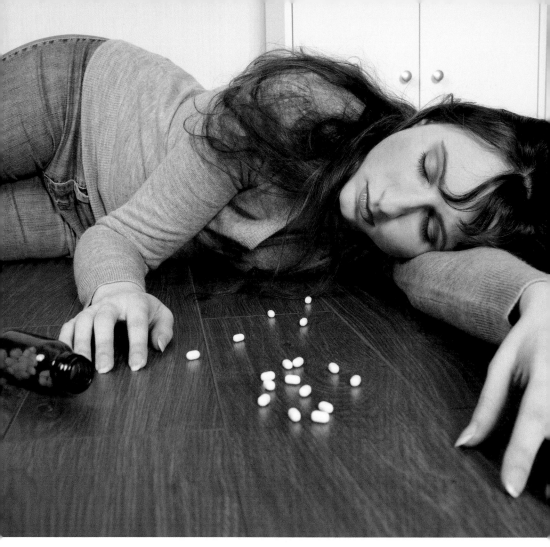

Tens of thousands of people in the United States overdose on drugs each year. That includes several thousand teens.

seizures. She called an ambulance. Kate was admitted to the hospital, where doctors confirmed she had overdosed on a legal, but unprescribed, drug.

Kate's parents could not understand how their active and vibrant daughter could be doing drugs. She was a high achiever. Now in her senior year, she was an honor roll student and captain of the volleyball team. She was set to attend college in the fall.

In Kate's case, they were lucky, and doctors got to her in time to save her life. Kate's parents would soon learn, though, that many are not so fortunate. Substance use disorder (SUD) is far more common than they knew. It tears apart families, destroys lives, and costs society billions of dollars. Kate is a fictional character based on a composite of real-life people. But stories like hers have become all too common.

A GLOBAL EPIDEMIC

In some societies it is normal for people to drink alcohol or smoke marijuana, and it is sometimes medically necessary for people to take drugs such as opioids or amphetamines. This kind of drug use occurs legally every day, and for many people it does not create a problem. However, some people, like Kate, develop an SUD.

The US National Survey on Drug Use and Health (NSDUH) is a research program directed by the US federal government. In 2018, it reported that 20.3 million people age 12 and older had an alcohol or illegal drug use disorder in the past year. Problems with substance use go beyond US borders. According to the United Nations Office on Drugs and Crime (UNODC) *World Drug Report 2018*, 31 million people worldwide struggled with drug

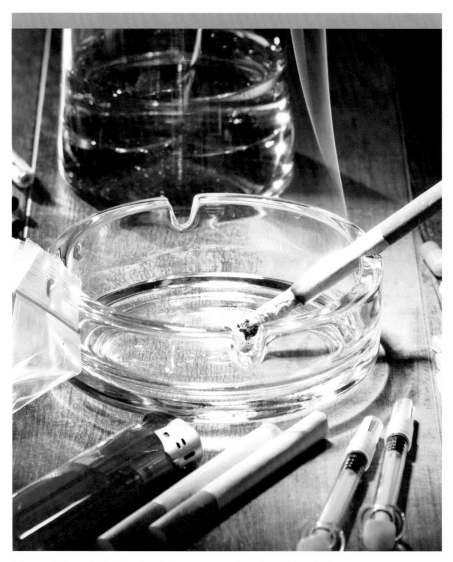

Many different kinds of substances are involved in substance use disorders. Some are legal for adults to use, while others are illegal for anyone to use.

use and 450,000 died from drug use in 2015. These numbers do not include alcohol.

As addiction researcher A. Thomas McLellan notes in a 2017 report, "These problems are not simply financial burdens—they deteriorate the quality of our health, educational, and social systems, and they are debilitating and killing us—particularly our young through alcohol-related car crashes, drug-related violence, and medication overdoses."[1]

> "These problems are not simply financial burdens—they deteriorate the quality of our health, educational, and social systems, and they are debilitating and killing us— particularly our young through alcohol-related car crashes, drug-related violence, and medication overdoses."[1]
>
> —Addiction researcher
> A. Thomas McLellan

CHAPTER ONE

What Is Substance Use Disorder?

SUD, often referred to as addiction, substance abuse, or substance dependence, is generally diagnosed by a medical professional when the patient continues taking a substance even though he or she knows it is dangerous to themselves or interferes with their day-to-day life. Medical professionals now rely on the *Diagnostic and Statistical Manual of Mental Disorders, 5th Edition* (*DSM-5*) to diagnose patients with SUD, but the guidelines have evolved over the years. The previous edition, *DSM-IV*, was used until 2013. The *DSM-IV* viewed this problem as a condition that progressed from substance abuse to dependence. The *DSM-5* introduced a new blanket term: SUD.

In his 2013 book *Clean*, journalist David Sheff describes the changes this way:

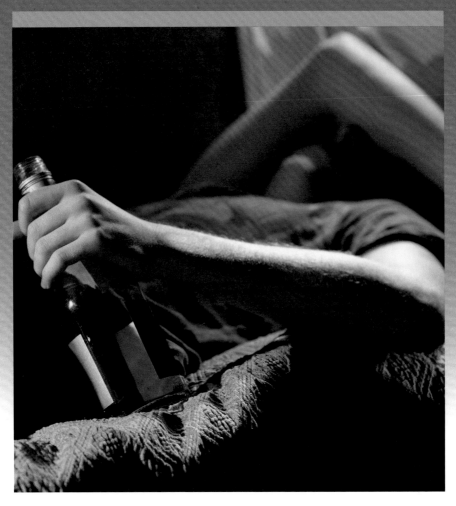

Alcohol use is common among people with substance use disorder. It can have short-term harm due to impairment, as well as long-term harm due to its other effects on the body.

The fifth edition of the DSM . . . essentially eliminates drug abuse as a stage separate from addiction. The new definition is nuanced but generally states that anyone who continues to use drugs in spite of harmful consequences has a substance [use] disorder and is an addict, on a scale from mild to moderate to severe. That is, addiction is a continuum that includes all persistent and dangerous use.[2]

WHAT IS A SUBSTANCE?

The "substance" in SUD can be either legal or illegal. According to the *Merck Manual*, an authoritative medical textbook, a substance usually falls within one of ten classes of drugs: alcohol; antianxiety and sedative drugs; caffeine; cannabis; hallucinogens; inhalants; opioids; stimulants; tobacco; and an "other" category, which includes anabolic steroids and other substances that create problems for their users.

These substances have a variety of mood-altering effects on users. They do, however, have similarities with regard to their effects on the brain. They affect the reward system in the brain, which for many people results in a sense of pleasure.

SUBSTANCE USE BY THE NUMBERS

Statistics demonstrate that people like Kate are not alone in their struggle. The NSDUH reported in 2018 that about 916,000 US adolescents ages twelve to seventeen had an SUD in the past year. Approximately 681,000 had a drug use disorder involving substances other than alcohol, and 401,000 had an alcohol use disorder. Many of those people struggled with both.

Older Americans experienced even more widespread SUD. Approximately 5.1 million young adults ages eighteen to twenty-five and 14.2 million adults ages twenty-six and older were also afflicted by an SUD in 2018.

ALCOHOL

Alcohol is the most common substance involved in SUD, though it is used more by older people than by teens. According to the 2018 NSDUH, in 2016 14.8 million adults ages twelve and older and 401,000 youth ages twelve to seventeen had an alcohol use disorder in the United States. These figures showed a significant decrease between 2002 to 2015, but they remained similar from their levels in 2016 and 2017.

Binge drinking, defined as drinking large amounts of alcohol in one sitting, is also a big problem. For men, binge drinking is consuming five or more servings of alcohol within the span of a few hours, and for women it is consuming four or more. The 2018 NSDUH reported that 67.1 million people in the United States were current binge alcohol users. Additionally, 1.2 million youth ages twelve to seventeen had engaged in binge drinking in the past month, and the majority of drinkers under age twenty-one said that they binge drink.

Although not all binge drinkers necessarily have an SUD, there are strong links between binge drinking as an adolescent and developing an SUD later in life. For example, one study showed a predictive link between binge drinking in grade twelve and SUD symptoms seventeen years later. Binge drinking has been shown to foretell midlife alcohol use disorders.

Alcohol misuse, like binge drinking, can lead to long-term health problems, including high blood pressure, heart disease, stroke, liver disease, and certain types of cancer, including breast cancer. It can also lead to unintentional injuries or deaths from falls, burns, car crashes, and alcohol poisoning. Between 2006 and 2010, alcohol-related deaths were the third leading preventable cause of death in the United States. The World Health Organization (WHO) reported that in 2010, alcohol misuse was the leading cause of death globally among people ages fifteen to forty-nine. One-quarter of all deaths for people ages twenty to thirty-nine around the world were attributed to alcohol.

PRESCRIPTION DRUGS

Prescription drugs are sometimes overlooked as potentially addictive because they are legal. People also might think these drugs are safer than illegal drugs because they are prescribed

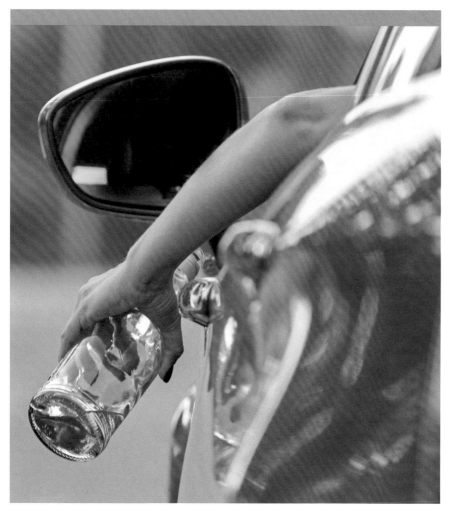

Driving under the influence of alcohol can have serious consequences for teens and those around them. Legal consequences, serious harm, or even death can result.

by a doctor. However, many legal prescription drugs are highly addictive and can cause just as many health problems for users as alcohol and illegal drugs.

The three main types of prescription medication that people misuse and become addicted to are opioids, which are often

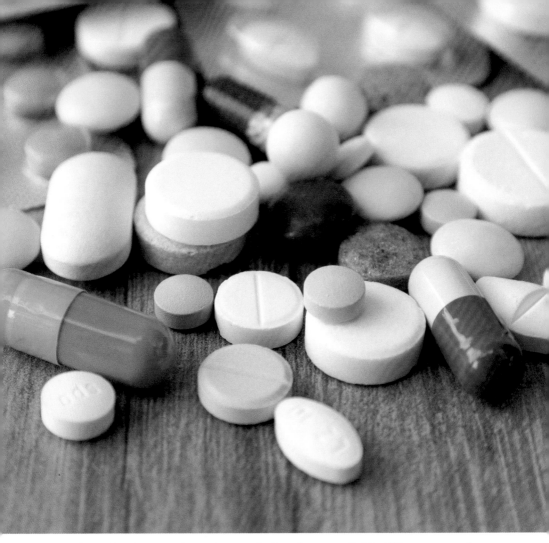

There is a huge variety of prescription drugs available. Whenever such drugs are taken without a doctor's prescription, there is the potential for serious harm.

prescribed for pain; depressants, which include tranquilizers and sedatives used to treat anxiety and sleep disorders; and stimulants, which are usually prescribed to treat ADHD. Each of these can have dangerous effects on the body.

Approximately 2 million Americans had an opioid use disorder in 2018. Opioids can cause drowsiness, nausea, constipation, and, if taken in large amounts, slowed breathing and death. Five percent of those with an opioid disorder will try the illegal opioid heroin, and 130 users die every day in the United States from an opioid overdose. Tranquilizers and sedatives can cause slurred speech, shallow breathing, fatigue, disorientation, and lack of coordination. Users may experience seizures when trying to stop use of these drugs. Stimulants can cause paranoia, dangerously high body temperatures, and an irregular heartbeat.

The 2018 NSDUH reported that 10.3 million people ages twelve and older had misused opioids, sedatives, or stimulants in the previous twelve months. Approximately one million people in this age category had misused prescription stimulants for the first time in the past year, including approximately 181,000 youth ages twelve to seventeen. This is an average of almost 500 youth who began misusing stimulants every day.

Misuse of prescription drugs is common in young adults, with 14.4 percent of people ages eighteen to twenty-five reporting past-year misuse in 2017. The 2018 Monitoring the Future survey, which examines drug use among eighth-, tenth-, and twelfth-grade students, found that 4.6 percent of high school students had taken Adderall for nonmedicinal purposes in the past year, and 2 percent had taken Vicodin, which is a combination opioid/nonopioid pain reliever. Approximately

60 percent of the respondents said they either bought or got the drugs from a friend or relative.

MARIJUANA

Cannabis, commonly known as marijuana, was long considered a dangerous and addictive drug with no practical medical purposes. It was made illegal in the United States in 1937. As a result, little research has been done on its effects on humans and society. More recently, however, attitudes toward marijuana have started to change. Most states have now legalized medically prescribed marijuana. Some states have also legalized recreational marijuana use, as have countries including Canada and Uruguay. With legalization increasing across the United States and around the world, some researchers predict that the number of users will increase.

The UNODC *World Drug Report 2019* estimated 188 million people worldwide used marijuana in 2017. The National Institute on Alcohol Abuse and Alcoholism (NIAAA), which studies a variety of drugs, has reported that between the periods of 2001–2002 and 2012–2013, the share of Americans who used marijuana increased from 4.1 percent of the population to 9.5 percent. Nora D. Volkow, director of the National Institute on Drug Abuse (NIDA), says, "These findings highlight the changing cultural norms related to marijuana use."[3] Dr. George Koob, director of the NIAAA, noted, "Based on the results of our surveys, marijuana use in the United States has risen rapidly over the past decade, with about 3 in 10 people who use marijuana meeting the criteria for addiction."[4]

"Based on the results of our surveys, marijuana use in the United States has risen rapidly over the past decade, with about 3 in 10 people who use marijuana meeting the criteria for addiction."[4]

—Dr. George Koob, director, NIAAA

Those listed as most at risk for marijuana use disorder were young adults ages eighteen to twenty-nine, with 7.5 percent meeting the *DSM-IV* criteria for a disorder, an increase from 4.4 percent over the past decade. It should be noted, however, that researchers attribute this increase to the overall increase in use, not due to an increase in rates of addiction.

The trend of legalization has medical experts concerned that people, particularly youth, will think marijuana is harmless and safe. The 2018 Monitoring the Future survey found that most twelfth-grade students did not view regular marijuana use as harmful. However, marijuana can be harmful. Volkow notes, "Levels of THC—the main psychoactive ingredient in marijuana— have gone up a great deal, from 3.75 percent in 1995 to an average of 15 percent in today's marijuana cigarettes. Daily use today can have stronger effects on a developing teen brain than it did 10 or 20 years ago."[5]

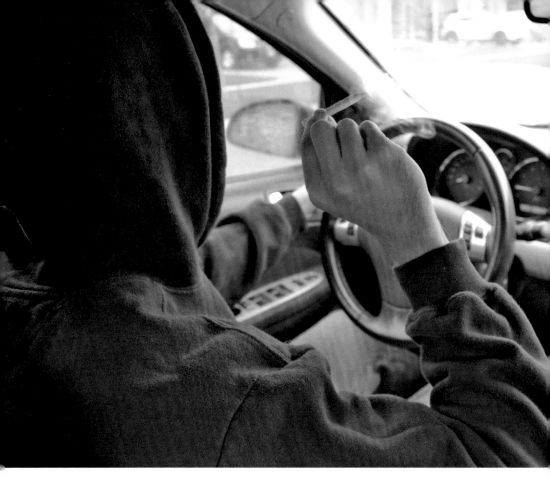

Marijuana has become legal in more places in recent years. However, it can still be harmful to teens, especially while doing activities such as driving.

Studies have shown that heavy use of cannabis during adolescence can inhibit the proper development of the brain, causing more severe and persistent negative outcomes than when use begins during adulthood. Some research indicates it is marijuana's effect on the endocannabinoid system (ECS) that interferes with proper brain development. The ECS, which helps the body respond to its environment in a variety of ways, was accidentally discovered while researching cannabis. Cannabis researcher Raphael Mechoulam explains, "By using a plant that has been around for thousands of years, we discovered a new physiological system of immense importance. We wouldn't have been able to get there if we had not looked at the plant."[6]

Everyone has an ECS, and it is active whether the person uses cannabis or not. More research needs to be done in this area, but so far researchers have discovered that the ECS is involved with regulating body functions such as sleep, appetite, memory, and mood. Researchers believe that using cannabis during adolescence, while the brain is still developing, can lead to future cognitive and emotional deficits because it interferes with the ECS.

Despite more widespread legalization and an increase in use among the general population, use among US high school students has not increased. The 2018 Monitoring the Future survey notes, "Daily, past-month, past-year, and lifetime marijuana use declined among 8th graders and remains unchanged among 10th and 12th graders compared to five years ago. . . . Past-year use of marijuana reached its lowest levels in more than two decades among 8th and 10th graders in 2016 and has since remained stable."[7]

ILLICIT DRUGS

Illicit drugs are those that are illegal to produce and obtain. There are four main types of illicit drugs: stimulants, such as cocaine and crack cocaine; narcotics, such as opioids; hallucinogens, such as LSD; and depressants, such as marijuana. Many of these drugs present multiple dangers. They have similar detrimental health effects as prescription drugs and alcohol, but they are produced illegally with no regulations, so unknown substances may be mixed into the drugs, increasing the risk of overdose and death. Also, because they are illegal, using, buying, or selling them comes with big consequences, including potential prison time, if a person is caught and charged with a crime.

Illicit drugs are often synthetic. This means they are made in a laboratory rather than occurring naturally. Synthetic opioids or cannabinoids are designed to mimic the effects of known legal

Needle Sharing and Disease Spreading

One of the most dangerous risks with substance use is the spread of preventable diseases from sharing the needles that are used to inject substances. HIV/AIDS and hepatitis C are the two most commonly spread diseases from this kind of drug use. HIV is a virus that attacks the cells that help the body fight infection and disease. This makes the person more vulnerable to those infections and diseases and can lead to a condition called AIDS. There is no cure. Each time a person uses a needle that has also been used by someone with HIV, the person has a one in 160 chance of getting the virus. Needles and syringes can get blood on them, and blood is what carries the virus. The virus can survive for up to 42 days on the used needle. Hepatitis C is also caused by a virus. It can lead to severe liver damage. Oftentimes people do not know they have it because it has few symptoms. However, it is very contagious and can spread through a small amount of blood. The most common way for people to acquire hepatitis C today is through sharing dirty needles.

drugs, but the chemical compounds are altered to get around illegal substance laws. They are usually manufactured outside of the United States and are much less expensive than their legal counterparts. They are still very dangerous. For example, one synthetic opioid, fentanyl, is partly responsible for the dramatic increase in overdose deaths in the United States and Canada in the 2010s. This drug, once only prescribed for cancer patients with extreme pain, started being produced illegally and sold on the street. It is up to fifty times stronger than heroin, and it is often mixed in with other drugs and consumed unknowingly by users.

Synthetic cannabinoids, unlike marijuana, are artificial products. They are sold in liquid form and are ingested using a vape pen or e-cigarette (electronic cigarette). The product is also sprayed on dried leaves so it can be smoked like marijuana. Synthetic cannabinoids are sometimes called fake weed or synthetic marijuana, but their effects are much more intense, unpredictable, and dangerous than those of marijuana.

VAPING

A new method of taking drugs that has become widespread among American youth is vaping. This is a method of ingesting nicotine or marijuana in aerosol, or vapor, form. It became very trendy in the late 2010s. Flavored oils are infused with nicotine or marijuana and heated in a battery-operated device until they become a vapor. Then the user inhales the vapor. There are a number of different names for vaping devices, including mods, vapes, sub-ohms, vape pens, e-hookahs, tank systems, e-cigarettes, and electronic nicotine delivery systems (ENDS).

Health care professionals are very concerned about this trend, as little research has been done on the effects of vaping on the human body. In late 2018, the US surgeon general, Jerome Adams, issued a rare national advisory on the subject. He said, "We need to protect our kids from all tobacco products, including all shapes and sizes of e-cigarettes." Adams added, "We must take action now to protect the health of our nation's young people."[8]

The Centers for Disease Control and Prevention (CDC), a US government agency involved in public health, also issued a warning that as of December 20, 2019, all fifty states and two US territories had reported 2,506 lung injury cases associated with vaping. Sixteen percent of the patients were under sixteen years old, and 38 percent were between the ages of eighteen and twenty-four. There had also been fifty-four vaping-related deaths. Dangerous chemicals had been found in the lungs of patients the CDC studied.

SUBSTANCE USE STATISTICS

The 2019 Monitoring the Future survey studied what percentage of high school students reported having used various substances in the past month.

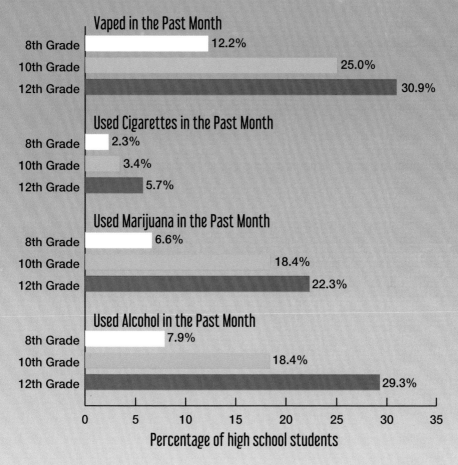

Vaped in the Past Month

Grade	Percentage
8th Grade	12.2%
10th Grade	25.0%
12th Grade	30.9%

Used Cigarettes in the Past Month

Grade	Percentage
8th Grade	2.3%
10th Grade	3.4%
12th Grade	5.7%

Used Marijuana in the Past Month

Grade	Percentage
8th Grade	6.6%
10th Grade	18.4%
12th Grade	22.3%

Used Alcohol in the Past Month

Grade	Percentage
8th Grade	7.9%
10th Grade	18.4%
12th Grade	29.3%

Percentage of high school students

"Monitoring the Future Survey: High School and Youth Trends," National Institute on Drug Abuse, December 2019. www.drugabuse.gov.

COSTLY ADDICTIONS

The costs of substance abuse are staggering. According to the NIDA, the combined cost of all crime, lost work productivity, and health care as a result of tobacco, alcohol, and illicit drug abuse is more than $740 billion annually. About $300 billion of that is related to tobacco. Alcohol has the next-highest share, at $249 billion, followed by illicit drugs at $193 billion and prescription opioids at $78.5 billion.

SUD is also impacting employment numbers. In a report released in the fall of 2017, Princeton University economist Alan Krueger reported that the opioid crisis could be responsible for up to 20 percent of the decline in male labor force participation and 25 percent of the decline in female labor force participation between 1999 and 2015. Labor force participation represents the total number of working people divided by the overall working-age population. In July 2019, testifying before the House Financial Services Committee, Chairman of the Federal Reserve Jerome Powell said that the opioid crisis is having a

"An extraordinary number of people are taking opioids in one form or another. It weighs on labor force participation, largely but not exclusively on younger males and younger women. It's a national crisis, really. The humanitarian aspect is completely compelling. But the economic impact is also quite substantial."[9]

—*Jerome Powell, chairman of the US Federal Reserve*

substantial impact on the economy. "An extraordinary number of people are taking opioids in one form or another," said Powell. "It weighs on labor force participation, largely but not exclusively on younger males and younger women. It's a national crisis, really. The humanitarian aspect is completely compelling. But the economic impact is also quite substantial."[9]

In July 2017, the *New York Times* reported that in Youngstown, Ohio, in jobs where a drug test is required, sometimes up to half the applicants failed the test. Situations like this are leaving employers short on workers. Michael J. Sherwin, chief executive of 123-year-old Columbiana Boiler, said, "Our main competitor in Germany can get things done more quickly because they have a better labor pool. We are always looking for people and have standard ads at all times, but at least 25 percent fail the drug tests."[10] A shortage of workers means that each year he loses $200,000 in business to foreign competitors because he cannot fill orders for the galvanized containers and kettles that Columbiana makes.

The impact on health care is also high. Dr. A. Thomas McLellan reported in 2017 that although only 8 to 10 percent of the general population have an SUD, 20 percent of primary care clinic patients, along with 40 percent of general medical patients at hospitals and more than 70 percent of emergency or urgent care clinic patients, are recognized as having an SUD.

CHAPTER TWO

What Are the Causes and Symptoms of Substance Use Disorder?

Diagnosing an SUD is the first step in getting help for the problem. Medical professionals rely on a standard set of criteria to make such a diagnosis. The *DSM-5* lists four general categories containing a total of eleven criteria for diagnosing an SUD. The first category of symptoms falls under the broad description of inability to control use. For example, these symptoms involve taking the substance for longer or more often than you are meant to, or wanting to use less but finding yourself unable to quit. They involve spending a lot of time and energy getting, using, or recovering from using the substance, and they involve the person craving the substance when he

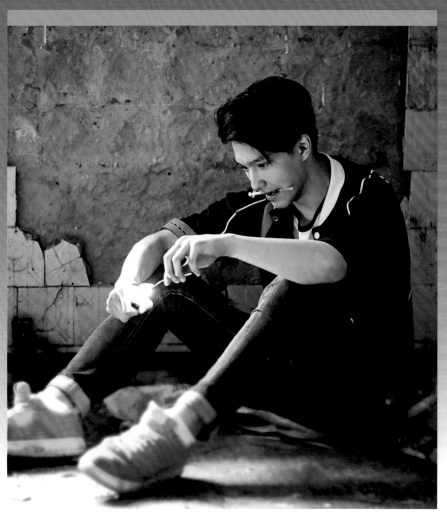

Continuing to use a substance even though you know it is harmful is a key part of substance use disorder. It is one of the criteria medical professionals look at when making a diagnosis.

doesn't have it. The second category relates to social symptoms. In these situations, using the substance is interfering with a person's social life, work, or school. For example, the person continues using the substance even though she knows it is causing problems in her relationships or is causing her to give up social, work, or recreational activities. The third category, risky use, includes using the substance continuously even if it puts the person in danger, or continuing to use it even if the person knows a physical or mental health issue could be made worse by using it. The final category of symptoms is physical. This involves needing more and more of the substance to get the desired effect and the person's body reacting negatively and craving more of the substance when he stops using it.

A person who presents with two or three of these criteria would be considered to have a mild disorder. Four or five criteria would indicate a moderate disorder. Presenting with six or more criteria would classify a person as having a severe SUD.

Sometimes people are diagnosed because they go to their doctor seeking help. It is more difficult to diagnose a problem if the person is trying to hide that they are using a substance. There are, however, some common signs of a problem. These signs include missing classes and wanting more privacy; being exhausted one minute, full of energy the next, and then defensive when asked about it; and spending more money than usual with no explanation for where the money is going. Such behaviors can alert people that a friend or family member has an SUD.

Stephanie King, the parent of substance user, explained in a blog post on drugfree.org the changes she saw in her daughter: "It was like a light switch—my beautiful, kind and sweet daughter was spending all her spare time isolating in her bedroom away from the family. She'd have random outbursts and treated me very poorly. I kept asking myself, 'Where did my daughter go?' It started to get really bad; worse than you could possibly imagine."[11]

WHAT CAUSES SUBSTANCE ABUSE?

Despite the fact that there are a huge number of people worldwide who use substances, only 10 to 20 percent of users develop an SUD. Medical professionals and researchers have struggled to understand why most people can consume substances occasionally and never develop an SUD, while for some addiction seems unavoidable. Kenneth E. Leonard, director of the Research Institute on Addictions at the University at Buffalo, New York, explains the complexity of addiction in a 2015 *Nature* article: "Addiction is more than a disease and involves more than the brain: it is a systemic behavioural disorder arising from and maintained by psychological, social, and biological processes operating both independently and in concert."[12] This makes it complicated both to diagnose and to treat.

> "Addiction is more than a disease and involves more than the brain: it is a systemic behavioural disorder arising from and maintained by psychological, social, and biological processes operating both independently and in concert."[12]
>
> —Kenneth E. Leonard, director of the Research Institute on Addictions, University at Buffalo

People often refer to the "addictive personality" as an explanation for why some people develop SUDs and others don't. However, addiction researcher Stephen Bright points out, "Personality is comprised of broad, measurable, stable, individual traits that predict behaviour. So, by definition, engaging in excessive behaviours cannot be considered a personality trait."[13]

Although Bright does not believe there is such thing as an addictive personality, he does think there are personality traits that correlate with addictive behavior. Bright details the five primary personality traits that drive behavior: openness to experience; conscientiousness; extraversion/introversion; agreeableness; and neuroticism. The last of those, neuroticism, correlates with addictive behavior. Neuroticism is a tendency toward a negative state. Neurotic people tend to be more depressed, and they often feel guilty, anxious, or envious. People who score high in neuroticism also are more likely to participate in excessive gambling, overeating, and substance misuse. Neuroticism has also been associated with other mental health issues, including emotional disorders and psychotic symptoms. Bright summarizes, "While there are common factors associated with personality that predict addiction, there is no personality type that will cause someone to partake in excessive behaviours. Addiction has multiple causes and just chalking it up to someone's personality probably isn't very helpful in dealing with it."[14]

Most experts do believe, however, there are three things that most influence whether a person will develop an SUD. The first is genetics. The second factor is mental health. The third is the person's environment.

Scientists have found that approximately 40 to 60 percent of the reason someone develops an SUD is genetic. Research has shown that children whose parents or close relatives are alcoholics are four to ten times more likely to become alcohol dependent than children who do not have alcoholic relatives. However, despite being able to link genetics in general to addiction, it has proven more challenging to link specific genes or traits to addiction. "What we're finding is that the addictive personality, if you will, is multifaceted," says NIAAA director Koob. "It doesn't really exist as an entity of its own."[15]

Some studies have shown a link between specific genes and specific addictions. A 2006 review of fifteen studies that included 4,500 Chinese, Japanese, Korean, and Thai participants showed that those presenting with the ALDH2 gene variant were nine times less likely to develop alcoholism than those with other

> "While there are common factors associated with personality that predict addiction, there is no personality type that will cause someone to partake in excessive behaviours. Addiction has multiple causes and just chalking it up to someone's personality probably isn't very helpful in dealing with it."[14]
>
> —Stephen Bright, senior lecturer of addiction, Edith Cowan University

variants of the gene. Another gene, CHRNA5, was strongly associated with cigarette addiction. Having just a single variant can double the risk of nicotine addiction.

People with an SUD also often have mental health problems. Mood and affective disorders, such as depression and bipolar disorder, are the most common co-occurring conditions. Patients often report using drugs or alcohol because they want to alter their mood. They are feeling depressed and want to feel happy, or they are feeling anxious and want to relax. In other words, their mood motivates them to reach for a substance in an effort to control and manage that mood. In the short term it feels like it's working, but over time the substance only degrades mood, and the same amount of the substance no longer has the desired effect. This leads to using more of the substance, which in turn degrades mood even more. The result is a cycle of behavior that worsens the disorder.

Like SUDs, mood disorders have a genetic risk factor. Perhaps not surprisingly, families with members who have a mood disorder are also more likely to have people who abuse substances among them compared to families without mood disorders. The coexistence of mental health issues and SUDs impacts the diagnosis and treatment of both. Missing a diagnosis of depression or bipolar in a person with an SUD could lead to more relapses and mood episodes, as well as a higher risk of

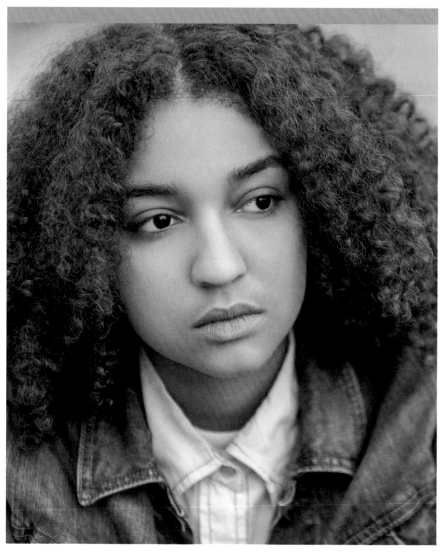

Substance abuse can interact with depression and other mental health problems. The intention may be for the substance to improve the mental health problem, but in the long run it can simply make things worse.

suicide. There is some research that shows treatment of one disorder can alleviate the other, and researchers are having some success developing methods to treat both disorders simultaneously. Still, more study is needed.

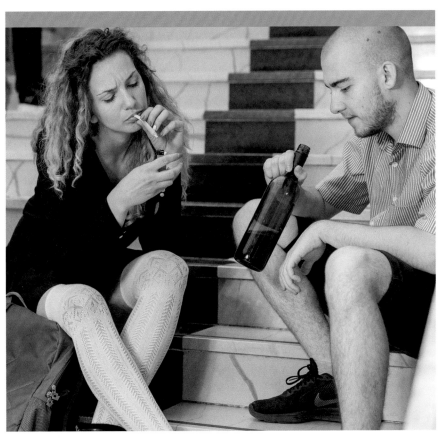

Peer use can lead people to use substances they might not otherwise try. The harm caused by substance use can spread through a group of friends.

A person's environment can also have an impact on whether they develop an SUD. Both their home and their broader environment, such as their neighborhood and even their whole city, can impact exposure to substance abuse. Environment can also affect their access to substances and treatment. If a person has environmental and social options for enhancing their positive moods and for coping with their negative ones, they are less likely to rely on a substance to help them cope. Likewise, if a person sees peers using drugs and alcohol as a coping mechanism, they are more likely to engage in similar activity.

Exposure to trauma has also been associated with SUD. One study of the Swedish population examined people who had lost their parents, people whose parents had been diagnosed with cancer, and people who witnessed domestic violence as children. These people had an increased risk of SUD compared to those who had not experienced trauma of this kind.

ABUSE LIABILITY

The concept of abuse liability refers to the potential a substance has for addiction and how drug manufacturers must take that potential into account. It is also referred to as "potential for addiction" and "addiction-sustaining properties." There is a requirement for drug manufacturers in the United States to determine the abuse liability of all new drugs they introduce to the market. Of course, this requirement does not exist for illicit drugs, but many have still been tested for it.

Abuse liability is measured using a combination of factors, including how the drug is used; how much it activates the brain's reward system; how fast it works; and whether it causes symptoms of tolerance or withdrawal. Heroin, cocaine, and alcohol often top the list of most quickly addictive substances.

Drugs with a higher abuse liability, whether legal or illicit, present a greater risk for developing an SUD.

Opioid Crisis

In 2017, the US Department of Health and Human Services declared a public emergency and developed a five-point strategy to combat the opioid crisis. The previous year, 42,000 people died from an opioid overdose in the United States, more than in any other year on record. The number of opioid deaths was six times higher in 2017 than in 1999.

The reason for the crisis has been largely blamed on drug companies that told doctors that opioids were not addictive and were safe to prescribe for pain. As a result, doctors started prescribing more of them. Sales of opioids skyrocketed in the two decades after 1999, increasing by 300 percent. In 2017, 191,218,272 opioid prescriptions were written by physicians. That figure was down slightly from the more than 200,000,000 issued yearly between 2006 and 2016.

Keith Humphreys, a drug policy expert, put the numbers into perspective: "Consider the amount of standard daily doses of opioids consumed in Japan. And then double it. And then double it again. And then double it again. And then double it again. And then double it a fifth time. That would make Japan No. 2 in the world, behind the United States."

Quoted in German Lopez, "America's Huge Problem with Opioid Prescribing, in One Quote," Vox, September 18, 2017. www.vox.com.

TOLERANCE, DEPENDENCE, AND WITHDRAWAL

When people use substances, they can build up tolerance to the effects. Tolerance means that a user needs more and more of the substance to get the desired result. People can build a very high tolerance to certain substances, such as opioids and alcohol, very quickly. Patients who are prescribed opioids to manage pain can develop tolerance in as little as a week.

Dependence occurs when quitting the drug causes the person to begin experiencing withdrawal symptoms. Some

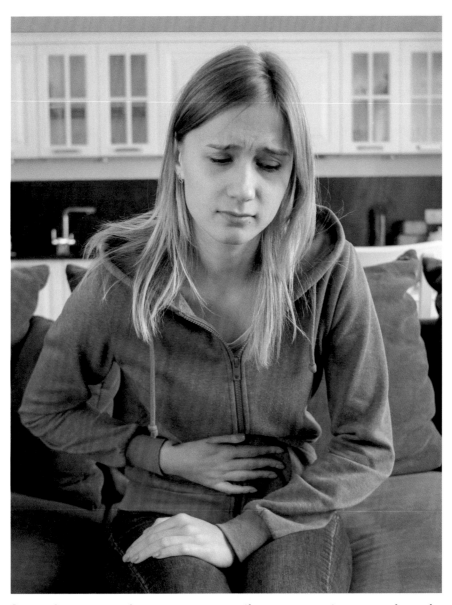

Stomach cramps and nausea are among the many symptoms experienced when going through substance withdrawal. Getting through this difficult period is critical in quitting a substance.

substances, such as caffeine, have relatively mild withdrawal symptoms. Others, such as heroin, alcohol, and opioids, can have life-threatening withdrawal symptoms.

Withdrawal is dependent on several factors, including how long and how frequently the substance was used, whether the person was using the drug recreationally or for medical reasons, and whether the person has a temporary dependence or a more severe SUD. Withdrawal symptoms are worse the longer someone has been using a drug. General symptoms of withdrawal can be broken down into four mental and emotional symptoms and six physical ones. Mental and emotional withdrawal symptoms include anxiety, depression, disrupted sleep, and memory and concentration problems. Physical symptoms include headaches and dizziness, tightness of chest and difficulty breathing, racing heart or skipping heartbeats, nausea and vomiting, muscle twitches and aches, and sweating and tingling skin.

Suicide and Substance Use

The *American Journal of Psychiatry* lists suicide as the tenth leading cause of death in the United States. Individuals with an SUD are ten to fourteen times more likely to die by suicide than the general population. Alcohol and opioids lead the way when it comes to deaths by suicide. Alcohol intoxication is involved in 22 percent of suicides, and opioids are involved in 20 percent. Marijuana, cocaine, and amphetamines round out the list of the top five. Using opioids is strongly linked to increased thoughts of suicide as well as a 75 percent increase in the likelihood of attempting suicide. Increased suicidal thoughts were also a risk for those who started drinking at a young age, binge drinkers, and for those meeting the *DSM-5* criteria for an alcohol use disorder.

Withdrawal from an opioid can be very unpleasant. Early withdrawal symptoms include feeling anxious and craving the drug. This is followed by rapid breathing, yawning, sweating, watering eyes, a running nose, and stomach cramps. People might become hyperactive or agitated, and their heart rate and blood pressure increase. Other symptoms include goose bumps, tremors, muscle twitching, fever and chills, and aching muscles. Withdrawal from an opioid can begin within four hours of the last time a person used the drug, but it usually peaks around forty-eight to seventy-two hours after that time.

Tracey Anne Duncan, a former drug user, described what opioid withdrawal feels like in a 2017 *Vice* article: "You want to know what it feels like? It feels like the worst flu you ever had, the sickest you've ever been, times suicidal thoughts and complete and total confidence that you are never, ever, ever going to feel better. It feels like the day your wife left and your kitten died and there were no more rainbows anywhere and never will be again."[16]

Withdrawal from alcohol can be quite intense and scary. Mild withdrawal symptoms include tremors, headaches, sweating, and nausea. Heavy drinkers can experience alcoholic hallucinosis, a condition where they see hallucinations and hear voices that seem threatening, causing apprehension and fear. The worst kind of alcohol withdrawal is delirium tremens,

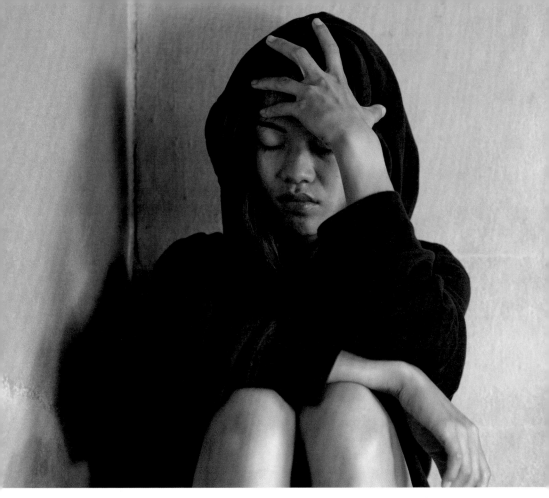

Alcohol withdrawal is a challenging time for someone with substance use disorder. The temptation to use the substance again can be strong.

otherwise known as the DTs. It usually sets in forty-eight to seventy-two hours after stopping drinking. It progresses from anxiety, confusion, and poor sleep to nightmares, excessive sweating, and depression. Blood pressure increases, the pulse rate goes up, and body temperature rises. Hallucinations and disorientation are sometimes terrifying. Balance is impaired, and confusion sets in, so the person thinks walls are falling or the room is spinning. Constant tremors occur that sometimes extend throughout the body.

Bestselling crime author Lowell Cauffiel described his withdrawal from alcohol in a *USA Today* interview as feeling like his "guts were being pulled out."[17] It wasn't until after he went through withdrawal alone that he found out doing so could have been fatal. It has been reported that as many as one in twenty-five people experiencing the DTs die. In the midst of all the suffering from withdrawal symptoms, people know that taking the substance again will relieve their symptoms. This is one of the greatest challenges those with an SUD face when they try to quit using substances.

CHAPTER THREE

What Is Life like with a Substance Use Disorder?

Living with an SUD is not easy on the user or those with whom the user interacts. Often it takes a long time before anyone notices that someone has reached the point of having a disorder. Over time however, chronic substance misuse inevitably impacts all aspects of a person's life, including health and hygiene; family and friends; employment and finances; and housing and security.

HEALTH AND HYGIENE

Both the short- and long-term health and hygiene of a person with an SUD suffer. Long-term substance misuse can cause dental problems, malnutrition, skin lesions, high blood pressure,

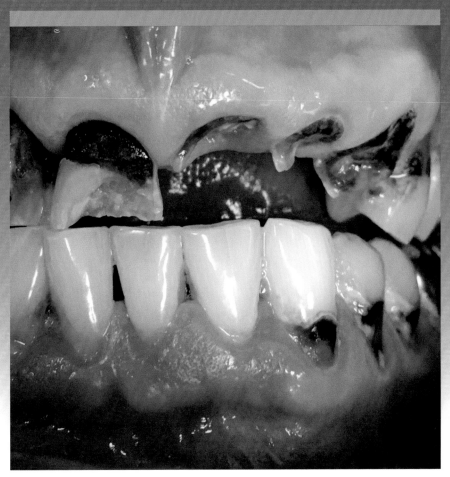

Using certain substances can cause severe dental problems. These issues can affect not only the mouth, but also other parts of the body.

heart disease, liver disease, kidney damage, injury, overdose, and eventually death.

Crystal methamphetamine, for example, rots teeth. Dr. Doug Bing is a dentist practicing in a suburb of Vancouver, Canada. His community has been adversely affected by meth use, and he says he has never seen anything like it in young adults: "The effect on teeth is similar to what we see in young children who have been put to sleep with a bottle of juice."[18]

Substance users often have dental problems for several reasons, including poor oral hygiene and a tendency to ignore symptoms due to the drugs dulling their pain. Drug users' teeth are also affected by excessive chewing, tooth grinding, and clenching. Also, saliva is a natural tooth protector, but using meth causes a decrease in saliva flow. This factor, combined with the dehydration also caused by drug use, leads to thirst. "Then they drink sugary soda pop to quench their thirst which only adds to the problem," says Dr. Bing.[19] All of this contributes to the deterioration of teeth.

> "The effect [of methamphetamine] on teeth is similar to what we see in young children who have been put to sleep with a bottle of juice."[18]
>
> —Dr. Doug Bing, dentist

Dental problems can lead to a myriad of health issues. The mouth is the entry point for both the respiratory and digestive systems. If bacteria are not controlled through good hygiene, they can reach a dangerous level and cause disease. Poor oral health has been linked to endocarditis, an infection of the inner lining of the heart chambers that can occur when bacteria from the mouth spread through the bloodstream and attach to parts of the heart. Periodontitis, the most severe form of gum disease, has been linked to heart disease, premature birth, and low birth weight. And pneumonia can be caused by bacteria in the mouth being pulled into the lungs.

There is also a strong correlation between chronic substance misuse and malnutrition. One study of alcohol- and opioid-dependent patients found that 24 percent of participants had mild or moderate malnutrition. Almost 90 percent of respondents needed nutritional advice and guidance from their doctor. Half of the participants were low in nutrients such as iron, potassium, and vitamins A and C. The researchers believed their results likely underrepresented overall malnutrition and its associated risk factors.

People who chronically misuse a substance are also prone to skin problems. These conditions are caused by several factors, including the substance involved, possible impurities in the substance, how the substance is consumed, and unhealthy eating, sleeping, and grooming habits. Compulsive skin picking; cutaneous abscesses, which are localized collections of pus in the skin; and cellulitis, a bacterial skin condition, are among the more serious problems. Chronic cocaine abuse, for example, can cause death of skin cells; a blackening of the palms; and a condition called Schonlein-Henoch vasculitis, in which blood vessels in the skin inflame and cause red spots that bleed.

Dangerous and Deadly

Experimenting with drugs, both legal and illicit, can be a dangerous game for people of all ages. According to the CDC, 70,237 people died in 2017 from a drug overdose. This represents an increase in the death rate compared to 2016, rising from 19.8 to 21.7 deaths per 100,000 people. The CDC also reported that 80.4 percent of drug overdose deaths in teens ages fifteen to nineteen were unintentional. In 2013, 12.4 people per 100,000 died from drug overdoses in the United States, compared to 2.5 people per 100,000 in similar countries. Opioids such as oxycodone, heroin, and fentanyl are responsible for the majority of overdose deaths, with 67.8 percent of drug overdose deaths in 2017 involving an opioid.

Alcohol is just as dangerous and deadly as other drugs. The CDC reports that 4,300 youth under 21 die from alcohol related causes each year. In 2013, 119,000 youth visited the emergency room for alcohol-related illness or injury. The CDC estimates alcohol and related causes account for 88,000 deaths every year in the United States.

FAMILY AND FRIENDS

Living with an SUD alters all of a person's interpersonal relationships. The nature of the disorder breeds mistrust because oftentimes users are trying to hide their problem. Sometimes, people start stealing to subsidize their addictions. In extreme cases, the disorder can lead to incarceration, which further alienates the person from family, friends, and opportunities. All too often, relationships are damaged and families are torn apart.

In a 2014 interview with CNN, Barbara Theodosiou described how she felt when she discovered both her sons were addicted to drugs: "I found out within six months that both my sons were addicts and like every other mother, I just wanted to go into bed and never get out."[20] Instead she went to

Facebook and started a page called the Addict's Mom. By 2019 it had more than 100,000 followers.

Theodosiou and the other mothers interviewed for the CNN profile all described being the mother of an addict as very lonely and said there is stigma associated with having a child with an addiction problem. "There are no little girls selling cookies for addiction," said Theodosiou. "Nobody has bumper stickers on their car."[21]

One of the biggest challenges the loved ones of an addict face is enabling. They want to be there to help their loved one, but sometimes their help only enables the person to continue using. Parents may

> "There are no little girls selling cookies for addiction. Nobody has bumper stickers on their car."[21]
>
> —*Barbara Theodosiou, mother of drug users*

make the difficult decision to walk away from their child rather than risk their own physical and mental health. It's "the hardest thing in the entire word," said Theodosiou. "All of these people were telling me you have to stop enabling Daniel. You need to let Daniel go. You need to just stop. . . . I had to actually face leaving Daniel on the street."[22]

Communities may reject people who abuse substances. Theodosiou explained one of her sons was in a church group.

She said, "When they found out he was an addict, the entire church shunned him. He was completely not invited anywhere."[23]

Another tragic social consequence of SUDs are children of adults with the disorder. These children have a much higher chance of developing an SUD. A 2013 study reported that adolescents exposed to parental SUD have an increased risk of developing one later in life. Many of these children are removed from their parents' homes or lose their parents to a drug overdose, and they frequently end up shuffled from foster home to foster home.

EMPLOYMENT AND FINANCES

SUDs can and often do interfere with future opportunities, including making it on a team, getting accepted to college, or getting and keeping a job. Since a 2002 Supreme Court ruling, schools are allowed to drug-test all middle and high school students participating in competitive extracurricular activities. The United States has very strict drug laws. If people are convicted of a drug offense, it can prevent them from getting jobs and joining the military, restrict travel, or even land them in jail and leave them with a criminal record.

An SUD can also have a profound effect on a person's ability to do their job and on the safety and well-being of their

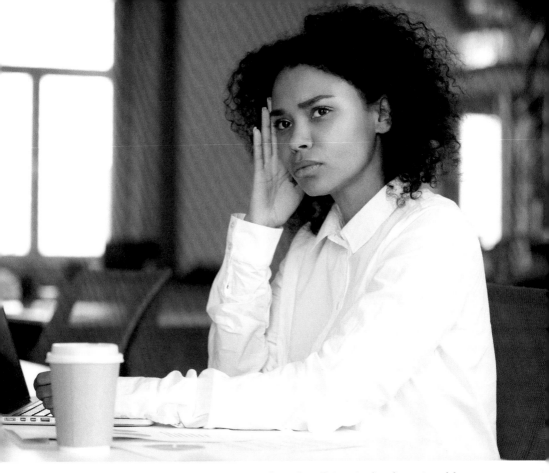

Substance use disorder can cause people to be distracted or have trouble thinking clearly at school or work. This can negatively affect their lives in many ways.

coworkers. The most common impacts at work are being late or absent due to a hangover or withdrawal; lack of alertness or awareness; being less efficient at completing tasks; and not getting along with coworkers. The National Safety Council reports that employees with an alcohol disorder are 34 percent more likely to miss work than those without, and they are more likely to be injured on the job. People with an opioid disorder missed three extra weeks of work per year compared to the general population. In many instances, a person loses their job because of poor performance.

Reporter Jayne O'Donnell described when she hit rock bottom by showing up drunk for her on-air job: "It surprised even me that I would drink all through Super Bowl Sunday, stopping only to sleep about an hour before showing up for a 6 a.m. TV spot the next day, Jan. 27, 1992."[24] After the taping, the producer told her he would make sure she never worked in Baltimore again. It took several dangerous accidents and the death of two friends due to alcohol before O'Donnell sought help and quit drinking. For those that are unable to do so, losing their job has dire financial consequences, impacting the person's ability to take care of themselves and often leading to further substance abuse.

HOUSING AND PERSONAL SECURITY

Another drastic consequence of an SUD is homelessness. Studies have shown that more than a third of people who are homeless are dealing with substance use problems, and up to two-thirds of them have had these problems at some point in their lives. Researchers note that substance use can not only cause homelessness, but also result from it.

Katie Kirkman, who works at a medical clinic for marginalized youth in Portland, Oregon, says that substance use can be one way that young people facing challenges try to make themselves feel better—though in the end it just makes their problems worse. She says, "Youth experiencing homelessness tend to have experienced significant trauma in their life and often cope through substance use, and also experience other mental health issues, like depression, anxiety, and psychosis, which are all further complicated by substance use."[25]

"Youth experiencing homelessness tend to have experienced significant trauma in their life and often cope through substance use, and also experience other mental health issues, like depression, anxiety, and psychosis, which are all further complicated by substance use."[25]

—Katie Kirkman, clinician at a Portland clinic for marginalized youth

CHAPTER FOUR

How Is Substance Use Disorder Treated?

People with SUD often face discrimination. In a 2017 article, *American Nurse Today* reported that a survey found that more than 50 percent of respondents believed treatment options for drug addiction were not effective, and nearly half the people were against the government spending more money on treatments. Additionally, while two-thirds of respondents said they did not think discrimination toward people with drug addiction was a serious problem, 43 percent were against equal insurance benefits for drug addiction, and almost 80 percent said they would not work closely with someone with a drug addiction. The authors go on to note that the stigma and stereotypes related to SUD may contribute to less than optimal care or create obstacles in providing care.

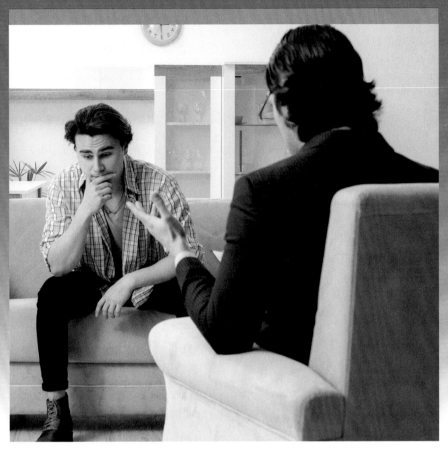

Counseling can play an important role in treatment for substance use disorder. It is one of the evidence-supported methods for overcoming this disorder.

Attitudes about SUD are, however, changing. Rather than shifting blame onto those who develop a disorder, more people are acknowledging that it is a multifaceted phenomenon that requires a multilayered treatment approach. Specific treatment strategies are dependent on the substance in question and whether the person has a mental health diagnosis. Usually treatment involves some combination of counseling, support groups, and sometimes alternative drug intervention.

Although researchers and clinicians continue to work on it, a perfect treatment has yet to be found. However, it is almost universally agreed among health care and treatment professionals that anyone struggling to overcome an SUD must have a good support system around them if they hope to succeed. This support can come from a professional such as a counselor or psychologist; community groups such as churches or youth centers; family and friends; or organized therapy groups such as Alcoholics Anonymous (AA) or Self-Management and Recovery Training (SMART).

PSYCHOLOGICAL AND PSYCHOSOCIAL TREATMENTS

People with SUDs also often have mental health problems. In order to have the best chances for recovery, it is important to determine whether a patient has coexisting disorders. Psychotherapy will help to ensure underlying problems are not overlooked. A psychologist or therapist can also help patients develop better stress-management skills, address the impact of relationships and social influences, and build and maintain the motivation to stay away from drugs.

There are several types of psychological treatments that can be used, including cognitive-behavioral therapy (CBT), motivational enhancement therapy (MET), guided self-change (GSC), and prize-based contingency management (CM). CBT involves talking with a mental health professional in sessions that are designed to help the patient become aware of the thought processes that lead to substance use. These discussions, along with readings and activities, are meant to help the patient adjust their thinking. MET is a kind of psychological counseling that is meant to bring about rapid change by making sure the patient is motivated to make that change, rather than by having them go step-by-step through a standard recovery process. With GSC, patients self-monitor their substance use habits and record high-risk situations they find themselves in. Once they have increased awareness about these habits and situations, they work with a therapist to find ways to make meaningful changes that help them stop using substances. With CM, patients are monitored very closely and then rewarded for good behavior. For example, patients might

Substance-Induced Disorder

Many substances are toxic. Over time, their effect on the mind can mimic other mental health disorders. This is called a substance-induced disorder. These disorders are independent of any other coexisting condition because all the symptoms are a direct result of substance use. In 2005, a document by the US Substance Abuse and Mental Health Services Administration listed nine substance-induced disorders: substance-induced delirium, substance-induced persisting dementia, substance-induced persisting amnestic disorder, substance-induced psychotic disorder, substance-induced mood disorder, substance-induced anxiety disorder, hallucinogen persisting perceptual disorder, substance-induced sexual dysfunction, and substance-induced sleep disorder. The potential to develop these disorders adds to the already severe risks of substance use.

be required to submit to a regular drug screening test. If they test clean, they are entered in a drawing to win money. This therapy is usually only used for eight to twenty-four weeks and in conjunction with other interventions such as group therapy. CM is most often recommended for people with cocaine use disorder.

For some people, the best course of action is to enter a rehabilitation center. Also referred to as residential treatment, recovery centers, or "detox" centers, these facilities can be perfect for people who want to achieve and maintain abstinence. Oftentimes familiar environments, family members, or peers can trigger relapses. The first twelve months after quitting a substance are the most difficult. Rehabilitation centers offer patients a controlled environment and a sober community. In addition to offering group therapy sessions and personalized drug and alcohol counseling, they also engage patients in basic care and maintenance duties, as well as off-site trips and activities. Patients benefit from living in a community and having social interactions with people they can relate to.

GROUP THERAPY AND TWELVE-STEP PROGRAMS

Twelve-step programs, including AA, Cocaine Anonymous (CA), and Narcotics Anonymous (NA), are among the most well-known group therapies. The only requirement for membership is a desire to quit using alcohol or drugs. In 2007, approximately five million people attended a twelve-step self-help meeting. About 45 percent did so for alcohol use, 22 percent because of illicit drug use, and 33 percent for a combination of the two. In 2012, there were an estimated 64,000 AA groups with 1.4 million members in the United States and Canada and an estimated 114,000 groups worldwide with 2.1 million members. The basic tenets are avoiding drinking and drugs, attending meetings, getting a sponsor, asking for help and helping others, and getting active.

A survey conducted by AA and NA found that respondents who reported attending two to four meetings a week had a median abstinence rate of greater than five years. Other studies support this, finding that participation in twelve-step programs is associated with longer abstinence as well as improved functioning and greater belief in one's ability to succeed.

Even those who have found success can be skeptical and wonder how and why the program works. Rae Steward, a recovering substance user from California, expressed this in an interview with Vox. "When I started doing the steps, I didn't think they were going to work,"

"When I started doing the steps, I didn't think they were going to work. I still, 10 years later, don't understand why they worked. But I feel like they gave me the design for living life. At this point, I just incorporate the steps in daily living."[27]

—*Rae Steward, recovering substance user*

she said.[26] "I still, 10 years later, don't understand why they worked. But I feel like they gave me the design for living life. At this point, I just incorporate the steps in daily living."[27]

Twelve-step programs aren't for everyone, though. Some people struggle with the idea of saying they are powerless, and some are uncomfortable with the religious or spiritual undertones. In the same Vox interview, Roger, who used a pseudonym for privacy, explained that after trying the program in 2012 and 2013 for drug and alcohol addiction, he was not able to stay with it. "I spent a year and a half staying blackout-ish drunk every night," he said.[28] He did eventually quit drinking in December 2014, attending some AA meetings and completing his twelve steps, but he did not stick with the program. Although he found the support of the meetings helpful, he has been able to stay sober without them.

For those who are looking for something other than the AA program, there are group therapies that aren't twelve-step programs. Over 90 percent of SUD treatment facilities offer some kind of group therapy, which can include skills training, motivational groups, educational presentations, or general check-in groups to hold patients accountable.

Therapies like SMART Recovery also follow defined guidelines to recovery. In the case of SMART Recovery, it is a four-point program that includes "building and maintaining

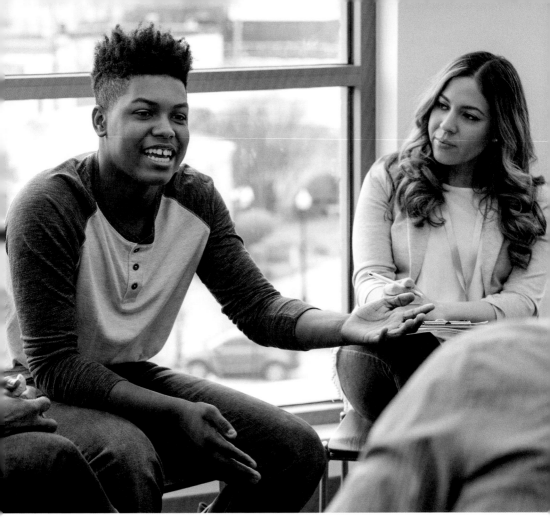

Group therapy can be an important part of SUD treatment. People can hear from others who have gone through similar experiences.

motivation; coping with urges; managing thoughts, feelings and behaviors; and living a balanced lifestyle."[29] The program features several tools and techniques for people to use and practice as they progress toward the final goal of the program. This aim is to achieve lifestyle balance and lead a fulfilling and healthy life. Some of the tools include worksheets to help people plan the change in their lives, worksheets to help people analyze the costs and benefits of their lifestyle, and methods of coping with urges. Whether it is a twelve-step program or another kind of group therapy, several methods involving therapy have been found to be effective in treating SUD.

MEDICATION-ASSISTED TREATMENT

For a long time, abstinence has been considered the gold standard in substance use treatment. Programs like AA are built on this foundation. However, Hazelden, one of the United States' largest chains of treatment centers, reported high dropout rates among those in opioid addiction treatment. Marvin Seppala, the group's chief medical officer, felt more needed to be done to improve this rate, stating in a 2015 *Nature* article, "We have to use everything at our disposal. We can't rely on a single approach."[30]

> "We have to use everything at our disposal. We can't rely on a single approach."[30]
>
> —*Marvin Seppala, chief medical officer, Hazelden*

Seppala believed medication-assisted treatment might help Hazelden patients stay in their treatment programs. He had seen a medication called Suboxone effectively reduce opioid cravings, and another medication called Vivitrol worked to block the effects of heroin and other opiates. However, using such medications was seen as contrary to Hazelden's abstinence approach. In 2012, he began holding information sessions with Hazelden staff.

"The use of a maintenance medication like Suboxone wasn't necessarily seen as appropriate," Seppala says.[31] "We thought they were going to throw tomatoes and rotten eggs."[32] This wasn't the case, however, and the treatment centers started offering Suboxone and Vivitrol to patients in combination with group counseling for opioid addictions. The results were promising. For those in the updated program only 5 percent dropped out in 2013 and 2014, compared to the previous dropout rate of 22 percent.

One medication-assisted treatment that has been used for a long time is methadone. Methadone is a painkilling opioid, but it is long acting, which means it releases more slowly into the blood. It lasts in the system for twenty-four to thirty-six hours, unlike other faster-acting opioids such as heroin, oxycodone, fentanyl, or hydromorphone. The effects of these drugs wear off within four hours, and withdrawal sets in. Methadone reduces cravings for the drug and prevents withdrawal symptoms. The purpose of replacing opioids with methadone is to stabilize people's lives and help keep them in treatment programs without relapse. When used for an opioid addiction, it is usually consumed in a liquid or wafer format and is taken once a day. When a doctor suggests a methadone maintenance program, it is not predetermined how long the treatment will last, but it is usually long-term and could last anywhere from one year to twenty years or more. Another drug that is used for medication-assisted treatment is buprenorphine. Although administered differently, its purpose and effects are like methadone. Suboxone includes buprenorphine as one of its components.

There are also medications effective in treating alcohol use disorder. Taken daily, disulfiram is prescribed to people who are alcohol dependent but have begun going through withdrawal. When taken with alcohol it causes physical reactions including nausea, vomiting, flushing, and heart palpitations. The awareness that these reactions are likely is meant to act as a deterrent to drinking. Naltrexone works in a different way. It blunts the rewarding effects of drinking. It can be administered as an extended-release injectable every four weeks, making it easier for patients to stick with their treatment. A drug called acamprosate affects the chemical pathways in the brain in a way that can reduce the cravings for alcohol.

SAFE INJECTION SITES

When it comes to SUDs, many people believe harm reduction is an important part of the treatment program. The goal with harm reduction isn't necessarily to get people to abstain from using a substance, but rather to use it in a safer way so they are less inclined to contract a disease or die from overdose. One harm reduction tool that has been used for those who inject drugs is

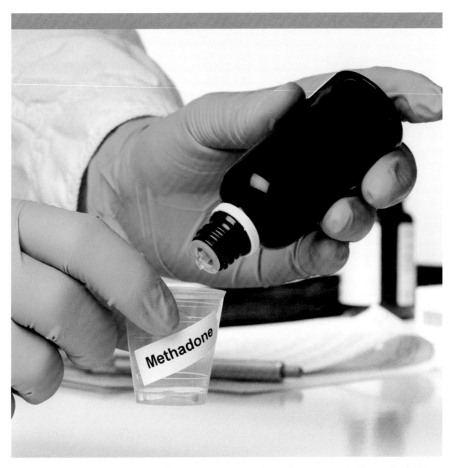

Methadone is one of several medication-assisted treatments targeted at a particular kind of substance use disorder. It is used to help ease users off of opioids.

safe injection sites. Also referred to as supervised consumption services, overdose prevention centers, supervised injection sites, and drug consumption rooms, they are legal facilities where people can self-administer preobtained drugs. They are meant to complement, not replace, other harm reduction, treatment, and prevention programs. Facility staff do not assist with drug consumption nor do they handle any drugs, but they are on hand to give out sterile needles, answer questions, provide first aid, watch for overdoses, and refer people for treatment. Australia, Canada, Denmark, France, Germany, Luxembourg, the Netherlands, Norway, Spain, and Switzerland have a total of approximately 120 of these facilities. Safe injection sites are not legal in the United States.

In a 2015 magazine article, Chris Beyrer, president of the International AIDS Society and director of the Johns Hopkins Center for Public Health and Human Rights in Baltimore, expressed support for making safe injection sites a basic part of public health in the United States. "The evidence is overwhelming that needle-syringe exchange and safe injection facilities work, save lives, are cost-effective, and prevent new infections," he said.[33] "So, of course, we are vigorously working on trying to move the bar from saying this can only be done in an emergency to saying this is a part of basic public health."[34]

Insite, the safe injection site in Vancouver, Canada, is one of the most studied health initiatives in Canadian history. There is ample evidence that safe injection sites are effective in achieving their intended goals of reducing high-risk HIV and hepatitis C behaviors; increasing enrollment in treatment programs; improving public safety by reducing public injections and disorder; and saving costs in disease reduction, overdose deaths, and emergency medical services.

Dr. MJ Malloy with the British Columbia (BC) Centre on Substance Abuse told a local news station that Insite is working: "In the first four years the facility was open, there were over 1,000 overdose events within the facility itself."[35] However, he added, "We found that rates of fatal overdose in the area around Insite declined 35 percent after the facility opened—versus 9 percent in the rest of the city of Vancouver."[36]

> "The evidence is overwhelming that needle-syringe exchange and safe injection facilities work, save lives, are cost-effective, and prevent new infections. So, of course, we are vigorously working on trying to move the bar from saying this can only be done in an emergency to saying this is a part of basic public health."[34]
>
> —*Chris Beyrer, president of the International AIDS Society and director of the Johns Hopkins Center for Public Health and Human Rights*

In 2017 the American Medical Association (AMA) voted in favor of launching pilot facilities for medically supervised safe injection sites. In a press release, the association explained its decision: "Studies from other countries have shown that supervised injection facilities reduce the number of overdose deaths, reduce transmission rates of infectious disease, and increase the number of individuals initiating treatment for substance use disorders without increasing drug trafficking or crime in the areas where the facilities are located."[37]

"State and local governments around the nation are currently involved in exploratory efforts to create supervised injection facilities to help reduce public health and societal impacts of illegal drug use," said Dr. Patrice Harris, chair of the AMA Board of Trustees and the AMA Task Force on Opioid Abuse.[38] "Pilot facilities will help inform US policymakers on the feasibility, effectiveness, and legal aspects of supervised injection facilities in reducing harms and health care costs associated with injection drug use."[39]

> "We found that rates of fatal overdose in the area around Insite declined 35 percent after the facility opened— versus 9 percent in the rest of the city of Vancouver."[36]
>
> —Dr. MJ Malloy, BC Centre on Substance Abuse

TREATMENT COST

Rehabilitation centers, medication-assisted treatment, and safe injection sites all have a cost. The question is whether the cost is worth it. Most experts argue yes, the cost of treatment is worth it, because the inevitable results and cost of not doing anything are much greater. The position of the National Institutes of Health (NIH) is that treatment reduces substance use and its associated health and social costs. It is estimated that there is a return of between four dollars and seven dollars on every dollar spent on drug treatment. When health care costs are factored into the equation, the return jumps to twelve dollars for every one dollar spent. Societal benefits include improved work productivity, fewer substance-related accidents, and fewer deaths by overdose. Reducing incarceration rates among drug users also has financial benefits. It costs $24,000 to keep someone in jail for one year, whereas methadone maintenance treatment for one year only costs $4,700.

SUD affects too many American households. Although some substance use issues are improving, others are getting worse. In 2018, a historically low number of high school students reported drinking alcohol. However, heroin use among young American adults ages eighteen to twenty-five doubled in the previous decade, and the rate of heroin overdose deaths nearly quadrupled. By recognizing the signs and symptoms of SUD, learning how it affects people's daily lives, and getting educated on the treatment methods, people can help themselves and their loved ones avoid and escape substance use disorder.

Source Notes

Introduction: From High Achiever to Substance User

1. A. Thomas McLellan, "Substance Misuse and Substance Use Disorders: Why Do They Matter in Healthcare?" *Transactions of the American Clinical and Climatological Association*, 2017, 128: 112–130.

Chapter 1: What Is Substance Use Disorder?

2. Quoted in "What Is Substance Use Disorder?" *Beauterre Recovery Institute*, September 28, 2018. www.beauterre.org.

3. Quoted in "Prevalence of Marijuana Use Among US Adults Doubles over Past Decade," *National Institute on Alcohol Abuse and Alcoholism*, October 21, 2015. niaaa.nih.gov.

4. Quoted in "Prevalence of Marijuana Use Among US Adults Doubles over Past Decade."

5. Quoted in "Sixty Percent of 12th Graders Do Not View Regular Marijuana Use as Harmful," *National Institute on Drug Abuse*, December 18, 2013. archives.drugabuse.gov.

6. Quoted in Martin A. Lee, *Smoke Signals: A Social History of Marijuana*. New York: Scribner, 2012. p. 208.

7. Quoted in Conor Friedersdorf, "Tucker Carlson's Monologue Insults His Viewers," *Atlantic*, January 6, 2019. www.theatlantic.com.

8. Quoted in Erin Brodwin, "The US Surgeon General Just Issued a Rare Advisory about E-Cigs like the Juul—Here's Why Vaping Is Dangerous," *Business Insider*, December 18, 2018. www.businessinsider.com.

9. Quoted in Berkeley Lovelace Jr., "Fed Chief Powell Says the Economic Impact of the Opioid Crisis Is 'Quite Substantial,'" *CNBC*, July 10, 2019. www.cnbc.com.

10. Quoted in Nelson D. Schwartz, "Economy Needs Workers, but Drug Tests Take a Toll," *New York Times*, July 24, 2017. www.nytimes.com.

Chapter 2: What Are the Causes and Symptoms of Substance Use Disorder?

11. Stephanie King, "How I Knew My Daughter Was Using Substances and in a Mental Health Crisis," *Partnership for Drug-Free Kids*, April 3, 2019. www.drugfree.org.

12. Kenneth E. Leonard, "Perspective: Beyond the Neural Circuits," *Nature*, June 24, 2015. www.nature.com.

13. Stephen Bright, "Is There Such Thing as an Addictive Personality?" *The Conversation*, October 1, 2019. www.theconversation.com.

14. Bright, "Is There Such Thing as an Addictive Personality?"

15. Quoted in Maia Szalavitz, "Genetics: No More Addictive Personality," *Nature*, June 24, 2015. www.nature.com.

16. Tracey Anne Duncan, "Quitting Opioids Cold Turkey Made Me Want to Die," *Vice*, November 27, 2017. www.vice.com.

17. Quoted in Jayne O'Donnell, "Quitting Alcohol Can Be Deadly: Hundreds in the US Die Each Year," *USA Today*, November 27, 2018. www.usatoday.com.

Chapter 3: What Is Life like with a Substance Use Disorder?

18. Quoted in Racquel Foran, "Tooth or Dare," *Maple Ridge-Pitt Meadows News*, n.d. www.mrtimes.com.

19. Quoted in Foran, "Tooth or Dare."

20. Quoted in Kelly Wallace, "Being an Addict's Mom: 'It's Just a Very, Very Sad Place,'" *CNN*, August 28, 2014. www.cnn.com.

21. Quoted in Wallace, "Being an Addict's Mom."

22. Quoted in Wallace, "Being an Addict's Mom."

23. Quoted in Wallace, "Being an Addict's Mom."

24. Jayne O'Donnell, "My 'Bottom' Was Being Drunk on TV. But I'm Grateful I Hit It Before I Killed Myself or Others," *USA Today*, November 22, 2018. www.usatoday.com.

Source Notes Continued

25. "Healing Hands," vol. 20, no. 2, *HCH Clinician's Network*, September 2016. www.nhchc.org.

Chapter 4: How Is Substance Use Disorder Treated?

26. Quoted in German Lopez, "Why Some People Swear by Alcoholics Anonymous—and Others Despise It," *Vox*, January 2, 2018. www.vox.com.

27. Quoted in Lopez, "Why Some People Swear by Alcoholics Anonymous—and Others Despise It."

28. Quoted in Lopez, "Why Some People Swear by Alcoholics Anonymous—and Others Despise It."

29. "SMART Recovery," *McCall Center for Behavioral Health*, n.d. www.mccallcenterct.org.

30. Quoted in Cassandra Willyard, "Pharmacotherapy: Quest for the Quitting Pill," *Nature*, June 24, 2015. www.nature.com.

31. Quoted in Willyard, "Pharmacotherapy."

32. Quoted in Willyard, "Pharmacotherapy."

33. Quoted in Ken MacQueen, "The Science Is In. And Insite Works," *Maclean's*, July 20, 2015. www.macleans.ca.

34. Quoted in MacQueen, "The Science Is In. And Insite Works."

35. Quoted in Ken Miguel, "Safe Injection Sites a Success in Canada," *ABC 7 News*, August 29, 2018. www.abc7news.com.

36. Quoted in Miguel, "Safe Injection Sites a Success in Canada."

37. "AMA Wants New Approaches to Combat Synthetic and Injectable Drugs," *AMA*, June 12, 2017. www.ama-assn.org.

38. Quoted in "AMA Wants New Approaches to Combat Synthetic and Injectable Drugs."

39. Quoted in "AMA Wants New Approaches to Combat Synthetic and Injectable Drugs."

For Further Research

Books

Tracy Brown Hamilton, *I Am Addicted to Drugs. Now What?* New York: Rosen Publishing, 2017.

Jennifer Landau, *Teens Talk About Drugs and Alcohol*. New York: Rosen Publishing, 2018.

Peggy J. Parks, *Teens and Substance Abuse*. San Diego, CA: ReferencePoint Press, 2016.

Jennifer Skancke, *Addicted to Opioids*. San Diego, CA: ReferencePoint Press, 2020.

Internet Sources

"Opioid Facts for Teens," *National Institute on Drug Abuse*, July 2018. www.drugabuse.gov.

"Rise in Prescription Drug Misuse and Abuse Impacting Teens," *Substance Abuse and Mental Health Services Administration*, August 2, 2019. www.samhsa.gov.

"The World Drug Report 2019," *United Nations*, 2019. https://wdr.unodc.org.

Websites

Centers for Disease Control and Prevention (CDC)
www.cdc.gov

The CDC is a component of the Department of Health and Human Services. Its website is an excellent place to find information about dangerous substances, facts and statistics about SUD, and the latest news about research and developments.

FightAddictionNow.org
https://fightaddictionnow.org

FightAddictionNow.org is an online community support group that provides information, resources, real-life stories, and more about addiction and treatment.

National Institute on Drug Abuse (NIDA)
www.drugabuse.gov

The NIDA studies the causes and effects of dangerous drug use. Its website features information about commonly used drugs, statistics about drug use, and the latest research.

Index

Index Continued

Image Credits

About the Author

Racquel Foran is a freelance writer from Coquitlam, British Columbia, Canada. She has authored several nonfiction titles for school-age readers covering diverse subjects, including organ transplants, robotics, and North Korea, among others. When she isn't writing, Foran enjoys tending to her little free library, painting, and walking her dogs by the river.